THE CACAO REVOLUTION

How This Superfood Is Changing the World

Asa Eccleston Kibilski

CONTENTS

Title Page

Copyright

The Sacred Bean: Cacao's Ancient Origins and Divine History   1

Empires Built on Chocolate: The Economics and Politics of Cacao   4

From Bean to Bar: The Art and Science of Chocolate Making   7

The Chocolate Conquistadors: Cacao's Journey to Europe and Beyond   10

The Chemistry of Bliss: Cacao's Mood-Boosting Compounds   13

Brain Food: Cacao's Impact on Cognitive Function and Focus   16

Heart Health Hero: Cacao's Benefits for Cardiovascular Health   19

The Antioxidant Arsenal: Cacao's Defense Against Aging and Disease   22

The Gut Feeling: Cacao's Role in Digestive Health   25

The Chocolate Rituals: Cultural Significance and Traditions   28

Modern Chocolate Movements: Fair Trade, Single Origin, and Bean-to-Bar   31

Cacao Ceremonies: Ancient Wisdom for Modern Healing   34

Chocolate Therapy: Indulgence for Mind, Body, and Spirit   37

Beyond the Bar: Creative Culinary Uses of Cacao   40

Cacao Beauty Secrets: Nourishing Skin and Hair   43

The Cacao Economy: Empowering Farmers and Communities — 46

Regenerative Cacao: Cultivating a Sustainable Future — 49

Cacao Activism: The Fight for Ethical and Sustainable Chocolate — 52

The Chocolate Connoisseur: Tasting Notes and Terroir — 55

The Future of Cacao: Emerging Trends and Innovations — 58

Cacao for Kids: Nurturing the Next Generation of Chocolate Lovers — 62

Cacao Recipes: Delicious and Nutritious Ways to Enjoy This Superfood — 65

Cacao Resources: Further Reading, Organizations, and Experts — 68

The Cacao Challenge: 30 Days to Transform Your Health and Happiness — 72

The Cacao Manifesto: Embracing a Chocolate-Filled Life — 75

THE SACRED BEAN: CACAO'S ANCIENT ORIGINS AND DIVINE HISTORY

The aroma of chocolate is a universal language of comfort and indulgence. It evokes memories of birthdays, holidays, and moments of pure pleasure. Yet, beneath the sweet allure of modern chocolate lies a rich and complex history that stretches back thousands of years, intertwining with ancient civilizations, mythology, and spiritual practices.

Long before chocolate became a global commodity, it was a sacred bean revered by Mesoamerican cultures. The cacao tree, Theobroma cacao, meaning "food of the gods" in Greek, was believed to be a divine gift bestowed upon humanity. Its fruit, the cacao pod, held precious seeds that were transformed into a bitter, frothy drink reserved for rituals, ceremonies, and elite consumption.

The earliest evidence of cacao use dates back to the Olmec civilization in present-day Mexico, around 1900 BCE. The Olmecs cultivated cacao trees and likely consumed cacao beverages during religious ceremonies and for medicinal purposes. The practice then spread to the Maya civilization, who elevated cacao to a central role in their culture and spirituality.

For the Maya, cacao was not merely a food or drink; it was a bridge between the mortal and divine realms. Cacao beans were used as currency, offered as tribute to rulers, and even buried with the deceased to nourish their souls in the afterlife. The Maya word for cacao, "kakaw," was synonymous with strength, power, and divine wisdom.

The Maya creation myth tells of the gods sacrificing themselves to create humanity from maize dough and cacao. Cacao was thus seen as the lifeblood of the gods, flowing through the veins of humanity. The Maya also associated cacao with the underworld, believing that the cacao tree grew from the heart of a slain god. This dual symbolism of life and death reflected the cyclical nature of the universe and the interconnectedness of all things.

Cacao rituals were elaborate and often involved bloodletting, fasting, and prayer. Cacao beverages were prepared with various spices, herbs, and chili peppers, creating complex flavors that were believed to enhance the spiritual experience. The Maya believed that consuming cacao could induce visions, connect them with their ancestors, and open their minds to divine wisdom.

The Aztec civilization, who rose to power after the decline of the Maya, also revered cacao. They adopted many of the Maya's cacao rituals and beliefs, further solidifying cacao's status as a sacred and valuable commodity. The Aztec emperor Montezuma II was said to consume vast quantities of cacao daily, believing it enhanced his strength and virility.

When Spanish conquistadors arrived in the Americas in the 16th century, they were initially repulsed by the bitter taste of cacao. However, they soon recognized its value as a currency and trade commodity. The Spanish brought cacao back to Europe, where it underwent a transformation. Sugar and other sweeteners were added to make it more palatable to European tastes, leading to the creation of the sweet chocolate we know today.

While chocolate's journey to Europe marked a significant shift in its consumption and production, the legacy of cacao's sacred origins continues to resonate. Modern chocolate makers and enthusiasts are rediscovering the ancient wisdom and spiritual significance of cacao. Bean-to-bar movements and cacao ceremonies are reviving traditional practices and honoring the cultural heritage of this extraordinary bean.

The story of cacao is a testament to the enduring power of food to connect us with our past, nourish our bodies and spirits, and shape our cultural identities. As we delve deeper into the world of cacao, we uncover a fascinating tapestry of history, mythology, and science that reveals the true essence of this sacred bean.

EMPIRES BUILT ON CHOCOLATE: THE ECONOMICS AND POLITICS OF CACAO

As the alluring aroma of chocolate wafted across continents, it wasn't just palates that were captivated; economies and political landscapes were transformed as well. The story of cacao is not just one of taste and tradition; it's a narrative of power, trade, and the rise and fall of empires.

In the 16th century, the Spanish conquistadors, upon their arrival in the Americas, recognized the economic potential of cacao. Initially met with skepticism due to its bitter taste, cacao quickly became a valuable commodity, serving as currency and a symbol of wealth among Mesoamerican civilizations. The Spanish, realizing its lucrative potential, established plantations in their colonies, exploiting Indigenous labor to cultivate and harvest the precious beans.

The introduction of cacao to Europe sparked a "chocolate craze." The bitter drink, transformed with sugar and spices to suit European palates, became a symbol of luxury and status. Monarchs and aristocrats indulged in elaborate chocolate rituals, solidifying chocolate's position as a delicacy for the elite.

The demand for cacao soared, fueling a global trade network. Cacao plantations proliferated across the Spanish colonies, particularly in regions like Venezuela and Ecuador. These plantations relied heavily on enslaved labor, a dark chapter in cacao's history that continues to cast a shadow on the industry today.

The economic impact of cacao extended beyond the plantations. European cities like London, Amsterdam, and Paris became hubs for chocolate production and trade. Chocolate houses emerged as social gathering places for the upper class, further fueling the demand and solidifying cacao's role in shaping European culture.

The cacao trade also had significant political implications. European powers vied for control of cacao-producing regions, leading to conflicts and colonial expansion. The Spanish, Dutch, and Portuguese empires all sought to monopolize the cacao trade, recognizing its potential to generate wealth and power.

The struggle for control over cacao led to the establishment of colonial plantations in Africa, particularly in countries like Ghana and Ivory Coast. These plantations, like their counterparts in the Americas, relied on exploitative labor practices, perpetuating cycles of poverty and inequality.

The economic and political power wielded by cacao continued to shape global events for centuries. The rise of industrialization in the 19th century led to the mass production of chocolate, making it more accessible to the general population. This democratization of chocolate further fueled the demand for cacao, leading to increased production and trade.

In the 20th century, the cacao industry faced new challenges. Fluctuations in global markets, political instability in producing countries, and the environmental impact of cacao cultivation all contributed to a complex and often volatile landscape.

Today, the cacao industry is undergoing a transformation. Fair trade practices, sustainable farming methods, and efforts to empower cacao farmers are gaining momentum. Consumers are becoming more aware of the ethical and environmental implications of their chocolate choices, demanding greater transparency and accountability from the industry.

The story of cacao is a testament to the interconnectedness of food, economics, and politics. It is a reminder that the choices we make as consumers have ripple effects across the globe. As we indulge in our favorite chocolate treats, it's important to remember the complex history and ongoing challenges that shape the cacao industry. By supporting ethical and sustainable practices, we can contribute to a more equitable and just future for all involved in the production of this beloved bean.

FROM BEAN TO BAR: THE ART AND SCIENCE OF CHOCOLATE MAKING

The journey of cacao from a humble bean nestled within a colorful pod to the smooth, decadent chocolate bar we savor is a fascinating blend of art and science. It's a transformation that involves centuries-old traditions, meticulous techniques, and a deep understanding of flavor profiles and chemistry.

The process begins with the cacao pod, a vibrant fruit that grows directly from the trunk and branches of the cacao tree. These pods, varying in color from green to yellow to red, contain the treasure within: cacao beans enveloped in a sweet, white pulp. The pods are carefully harvested, typically by hand, using machetes or specialized tools.

Once harvested, the pods are opened, revealing the precious beans. The beans, along with the pulp, are scooped out and placed in wooden boxes or on banana leaves for fermentation. This crucial step, lasting several days, initiates a series of chemical reactions that unlock the complex flavors of cacao.

During fermentation, natural yeasts and bacteria break down the sugars in the pulp, producing heat and acids. This process eliminates the bitterness of the beans and develops the chocolatey notes we associate with cacao. The beans are turned and aerated regularly to ensure even fermentation and prevent mold growth.

After fermentation, the beans are spread out to dry under the sun. This drying process, which can take several days to weeks, reduces the moisture content of the beans and further develops their flavor. The beans are raked and turned frequently to ensure even drying and prevent spoilage.

Once dried, the beans are sorted and graded based on quality and size. They are then roasted to enhance their flavor and aroma. Roasting temperatures and durations vary depending on the desired flavor profile and type of chocolate being made. This step is crucial in bringing out the unique characteristics of each cacao variety.

After roasting, the beans are cracked and winnowed to remove the outer shells, leaving behind the cacao nibs. These nibs, the heart of the cacao bean, are then ground into a thick paste called chocolate liquor. This liquor contains both cocoa solids and cocoa butter, the two main components of chocolate.

The chocolate liquor is then conched, a process of continuous mixing and aerating that refines the texture and flavor of the chocolate. Conching can last from hours to days, depending on the desired quality and type of chocolate. This step removes any remaining volatile acids and harsh flavors, resulting in a smoother, mellower chocolate.

At this stage, additional ingredients like sugar, milk powder (for milk chocolate), and vanilla are added. The mixture is then tempered, a process of carefully heating and cooling the chocolate to stabilize the cocoa butter crystals and create a glossy finish and satisfying snap.

Finally, the chocolate is molded into bars, filled with various ingredients, or used in other confections. The possibilities are endless, ranging from simple dark chocolate bars to elaborate bonbons and truffles.

The art of chocolate making lies in the ability to balance science and creativity. Each step in the process requires precision and attention to detail, while also allowing for experimentation and innovation. Chocolate makers often develop unique recipes and techniques, highlighting the diverse flavors and characteristics of cacao beans from different origins.

The science behind chocolate making is equally fascinating. The chemical reactions that occur during fermentation, roasting, and conching are complex and nuanced. Understanding these processes allows chocolate makers to control and manipulate flavor profiles, creating a wide range of chocolate experiences.

From bean to bar, the journey of cacao is a testament to human ingenuity and the enduring allure of chocolate. It's a story that spans centuries, continents, and cultures, uniting us in our shared love for this decadent treat. Whether you're a casual chocolate lover or a passionate connoisseur, understanding the process behind chocolate making deepens our appreciation for the artistry and craftsmanship that goes into every delicious bite.

THE CHOCOLATE CONQUISTADORS: CACAO'S JOURNEY TO EUROPE AND BEYOND

The sweet symphony of chocolate as we know it today would not exist without a pivotal chapter in history—the introduction of cacao to Europe by Spanish conquistadors. This marked a turning point in the global narrative of cacao, forever changing its consumption, production, and cultural significance.

When Hernán Cortés and his Spanish conquistadors first encountered cacao in the early 16th century during their conquest of the Aztec Empire, they were met with a bitter, unfamiliar beverage. The xocolatl, as it was called by the Aztecs, was a frothy concoction made from roasted cacao beans, water, chili peppers, and various spices. It was not an immediate hit with the Europeans, who found its taste unpleasant and its texture unfamiliar.

However, the conquistadors quickly recognized the cultural and economic significance of cacao in Mesoamerican society. They observed how cacao beans were used as currency, offered as tribute to rulers, and consumed during sacred rituals. Intrigued by its potential value, Cortés and his men brought cacao beans back to Spain as a curiosity and potential commodity.

Upon its arrival in Europe, cacao underwent a transformation. The Spanish, accustomed to sweeter flavors, experimented with adding sugar, cinnamon, and other spices to the bitter xocolatl. This marked the birth of a new kind of chocolate—a sweeter, more palatable version that quickly gained popularity among the European elite.

Initially, chocolate remained a luxury item reserved for the nobility and wealthy merchants. Elaborate chocolate houses sprang up in major cities, offering a space for the upper class to indulge in this exotic new beverage. Chocolate became a symbol of status and sophistication, further fueling the demand for cacao.

As the popularity of chocolate spread throughout Europe, the demand for cacao skyrocketed. The Spanish, eager to capitalize on this lucrative market, established vast plantations in their colonies in the Americas, particularly in regions like Venezuela, Ecuador, and the Caribbean. These plantations relied heavily on enslaved labor, a dark chapter in cacao's history that continues to haunt the industry today.

The Spanish initially held a monopoly on the cacao trade, but other European powers soon recognized its potential. The Dutch, French, and British all sought to establish their own cacao plantations and trade routes. This led to fierce competition and even conflict as European empires vied for control of this valuable commodity.

The cacao trade also played a significant role in the colonization of other parts of the world. The Portuguese introduced cacao to their colonies in Africa, particularly in São Tomé and Príncipe, where it thrived in the tropical climate. Cacao plantations also emerged in other parts of Africa, Asia, and Oceania, further expanding the global reach of this once-obscure bean.

The introduction of cacao to Europe sparked a culinary revolution. Chocolate, initially consumed as a beverage, gradually evolved into a variety of forms. Chocolate bars, candies, pastries, and desserts emerged, tantalizing the taste buds of people across continents.

The cultural significance of chocolate also evolved. It became associated with celebrations, romance, and indulgence. Chocolate gifts became a way to express love and affection, and chocolate confections were often given as tokens of appreciation and gratitude.

The journey of cacao from the Americas to Europe and beyond is a story of cultural exchange, economic ambition, and the enduring power of taste. It's a reminder that food can transcend borders, shape identities, and influence global events.

As we savor our favorite chocolate treats today, it's important to remember the complex history that brought cacao to our shores. From the ancient rituals of Mesoamerican civilizations to the bustling chocolate houses of Europe, cacao has left an indelible mark on our world. And as we continue to explore the diverse flavors and possibilities of chocolate, we honor the legacy of the chocolate conquistadors who first introduced this extraordinary bean to the world.

THE CHEMISTRY OF BLISS: CACAO'S MOOD-BOOSTING COMPOUNDS

When you take a bite of rich, dark chocolate and feel a wave of pleasure wash over you, it's not just your taste buds celebrating – your brain is throwing a party too. Cacao, the raw ingredient in chocolate, is a treasure trove of natural compounds that work synergistically to uplift your mood and create a sense of well-being. Let's dive into the fascinating chemistry behind this delicious phenomenon.

Theobromine: Cacao's Gentle Stimulant

At the heart of cacao's mood-enhancing properties lies theobromine, a mild stimulant that's similar to caffeine but with a gentler, longer-lasting effect. Unlike caffeine, which can cause jitters and a sudden crash, theobromine provides a sustained energy boost without the unwanted side effects. It works by stimulating the central nervous system, increasing alertness and focus. Theobromine also dilates blood vessels, which can improve blood flow and oxygen delivery to the brain, further enhancing cognitive function.

Phenylethylamine (PEA): The Love Chemical

Cacao is also a rich source of phenylethylamine (PEA), a neurotransmitter that's often referred to as the "love chemical." PEA is released in the brain when we experience feelings of attraction, excitement, and joy. It triggers the release of endorphins, our body's natural painkillers, and dopamine, a neurotransmitter associated with pleasure and reward. Studies have shown that consuming cacao can increase PEA levels in the brain, potentially explaining why chocolate is often associated with feelings of happiness and romance.

Anandamide: The Bliss Molecule

Anandamide, another key player in cacao's chemistry of bliss, is a neurotransmitter that's naturally produced in our bodies. It's often referred to as the "bliss molecule" due to its ability to bind to the same receptors in the brain as THC, the psychoactive compound in marijuana. However, unlike THC, anandamide produces a milder, more subtle effect. It's been linked to feelings of relaxation, euphoria, and pain reduction. Cacao contains compounds that inhibit the breakdown of anandamide in the brain, allowing its effects to last longer and potentially contributing to the sense of well-being associated with chocolate consumption.

Tryptophan and Serotonin: The Happiness Boosters

Cacao also contains tryptophan, an amino acid that's a precursor to serotonin, a neurotransmitter that plays a crucial role in regulating mood, sleep, and appetite. Serotonin is often referred to as the "happiness hormone" because it promotes feelings of calmness, contentment, and well-being. Studies have shown that consuming cacao can increase serotonin levels in the brain, potentially explaining why chocolate is often used as a comfort food.

Flavonoids: The Antioxidants for Brain Health

Cacao is packed with flavonoids, a type of antioxidant that's been linked to numerous health benefits, including improved heart health and cognitive function. Flavonoids are believed to protect the brain from oxidative stress and inflammation, which can contribute to neurodegenerative diseases like Alzheimer's and Parkinson's. Research suggests that consuming cacao may improve blood flow to the brain, enhance memory and learning, and even boost mood.

The synergistic effect: It's all about the balance

While each of these compounds plays a role in cacao's mood-boosting effects, it's important to note that their combined action is likely what creates the unique and complex experience of chocolate-induced bliss. Theobromine provides a gentle energy boost, PEA triggers the release of endorphins and dopamine, anandamide induces relaxation and euphoria, tryptophan boosts serotonin levels, and flavonoids protect the brain. This symphony of neurotransmitters and antioxidants working together is what makes cacao such a powerful mood enhancer.

So, the next time you indulge in a piece of chocolate, remember that you're not just satisfying your sweet tooth – you're also nourishing your brain and promoting a sense of well-being. It's a delicious reminder that happiness can be found in the most unexpected places, even in the chemistry of a humble bean.

BRAIN FOOD: CACAO'S IMPACT ON COGNITIVE FUNCTION AND FOCUS

The notion of "brain food" may conjure images of complex supplements or obscure ingredients, but the truth is, one of nature's most delicious offerings also happens to be a potent brain booster. Cacao, the foundation of our beloved chocolate, has been shown to enhance cognitive function, sharpen focus, and even promote long-term brain health.

The Power of Flavanols: Boosting Blood Flow and Brain Function

Cacao's cognitive benefits are largely attributed to its rich concentration of flavanols, a type of flavonoid found in plants. Flavanols are powerful antioxidants that have been shown to improve blood flow to the brain, a crucial factor in cognitive performance. By increasing blood flow, flavanols deliver more oxygen and nutrients to brain cells, enhancing their function and promoting communication between neurons. This improved circulation has been linked to enhanced memory, attention, and overall cognitive processing speed.

Studies have shown that consuming flavanol-rich cacao can lead to significant improvements in cognitive function. In one study, participants who consumed a flavanol-rich cocoa drink daily for three months showed improvements in memory tests compared to those who consumed a low-flavanol drink. Other research has found that flavanols can enhance cognitive flexibility, the ability to switch between tasks and adapt to changing situations.

Protecting the Brain: Cacao's Antioxidant and Anti-Inflammatory Effects

In addition to boosting blood flow, flavanols also protect

the brain from damage caused by oxidative stress and inflammation. Oxidative stress is a process in which free radicals, unstable molecules that damage cells, accumulate in the body. Inflammation is the body's natural response to injury or infection, but chronic inflammation can damage brain cells and contribute to cognitive decline. Flavanols have been shown to neutralize free radicals and reduce inflammation, potentially protecting the brain from age-related cognitive decline and neurodegenerative diseases like Alzheimer's and Parkinson's.

Theobromine and Caffeine: Enhancing Alertness and Focus

Cacao also contains theobromine and caffeine, two mild stimulants that can enhance alertness and focus. While theobromine has a gentler, longer-lasting effect than caffeine, both compounds work by blocking adenosine receptors in the brain. Adenosine is a neurotransmitter that promotes sleepiness and relaxation. By blocking adenosine receptors, theobromine and caffeine can increase alertness, reduce fatigue, and improve concentration.

Theobromine has also been shown to improve mood and reduce anxiety, which can further enhance cognitive performance. Studies have found that consuming theobromine can lead to feelings of calmness and well-being, potentially reducing distractions and improving focus.

Magnesium: The Memory Mineral

Cacao is a good source of magnesium, a mineral that plays a crucial role in brain function. Magnesium is involved in over 300 biochemical reactions in the body, including those that support memory and learning. It helps regulate neurotransmitters, maintain healthy brain cell function, and protect the brain from damage. Research suggests that magnesium deficiency can impair cognitive function, while adequate magnesium intake may improve memory and learning abilities.

Cacao: A Multifaceted Brain Booster

Cacao's impact on cognitive function is not limited to a single mechanism. It works through a variety of pathways, including improved blood flow, antioxidant and anti-inflammatory effects, and the modulation of neurotransmitters. This multifaceted approach makes cacao a promising natural remedy for enhancing brain health and cognitive performance.

While more research is needed to fully understand the complex relationship between cacao and brain function, the existing evidence suggests that incorporating cacao into your diet may be a delicious and effective way to boost your brainpower. So, the next time you reach for a chocolate bar, remember that you're not just indulging in a sweet treat – you're also nourishing your brain and investing in your long-term cognitive health.

HEART HEALTH HERO: CACAO'S BENEFITS FOR CARDIOVASCULAR HEALTH

While often associated with indulgence and pleasure, cacao, the raw ingredient in chocolate, is proving to be more than just a treat for the taste buds. Emerging research suggests that this ancient superfood might also be a powerful ally in the fight against heart disease, the leading cause of death worldwide.

Flavanols: Nature's Blood Pressure Regulators

Cacao's cardiovascular benefits are largely attributed to its high concentration of flavanols, the same compounds responsible for its cognitive-enhancing effects. Flavanols have been shown to promote heart health in several ways, one of the most significant being their ability to improve blood pressure. Studies have consistently demonstrated that regular consumption of flavanol-rich cacao can lead to significant reductions in both systolic and diastolic blood pressure. This is due to flavanols' ability to increase nitric oxide production in the body. Nitric oxide is a molecule that relaxes blood vessels, allowing blood to flow more freely and reducing the strain on the heart.

Improving Blood Vessel Function: The Key to a Healthy Heart

Another way flavanols benefit heart health is by improving the function of blood vessels. They do this by increasing the production of a molecule called endothelium-derived relaxing factor (EDRF). EDRF, like nitric oxide, helps blood vessels relax and expand, further reducing blood pressure and improving circulation. Additionally, flavanols have been shown to reduce inflammation in blood vessels, which can contribute to the development of atherosclerosis, a condition in which plaque builds up in the arteries, restricting blood flow. By reducing inflammation, flavanols can help prevent the formation of plaque and lower the risk of heart attacks and strokes.

Cholesterol Management: Lowering the Bad, Raising the Good

Cacao's cardiovascular benefits extend beyond blood pressure and blood vessel function. Studies have also shown that it can positively impact cholesterol levels. Specifically, cacao consumption has been associated with a decrease in LDL cholesterol (the "bad" cholesterol) and an increase in HDL cholesterol (the "good" cholesterol). LDL cholesterol can contribute to the buildup of plaque in arteries, while HDL cholesterol helps remove excess cholesterol from the bloodstream. By improving cholesterol levels, cacao can further reduce the risk of cardiovascular disease.

Platelet Function: Preventing Blood Clots

In addition to its effects on blood pressure, blood vessel function, and cholesterol, cacao has also been shown to improve platelet function. Platelets are blood cells that play a crucial role in blood clotting. While clotting is necessary to stop bleeding, excessive clotting can lead to the formation of dangerous blood clots that can block blood flow to the heart or brain, causing heart attacks or strokes. Cacao contains compounds that can inhibit platelet aggregation, the process by which platelets clump together to form clots. By reducing platelet aggregation, cacao may help prevent the formation of harmful blood clots and reduce the risk of cardiovascular events.

More than just a treat: Cacao's Holistic Approach to Heart Health

Cacao's benefits for heart health are not limited to a single mechanism. It works through multiple pathways, including improving blood pressure, blood vessel function, cholesterol levels, and platelet function. This multifaceted approach makes cacao a promising natural remedy for preventing and managing cardiovascular disease. While more research is needed to fully understand the complex relationship between cacao and heart health, the existing evidence suggests that incorporating cacao into your diet may be a delicious and effective way to protect your heart.

However, it's important to note that not all chocolate is created equal. The cardiovascular benefits of cacao are most pronounced in dark chocolate with a high percentage of cacao solids (70% or higher). Milk chocolate and white chocolate, which contain less cacao and more sugar and fat, may not offer the same heart-healthy benefits.

So, the next time you reach for a piece of chocolate, choose dark chocolate with a high cacao content, and savor the knowledge that you're not just indulging in a sweet treat – you're also nourishing your heart and protecting your cardiovascular health.

THE ANTIOXIDANT ARSENAL: CACAO'S DEFENSE AGAINST AGING AND DISEASE

In the realm of superfoods, cacao stands tall, not just for its delightful taste and mood-boosting properties but also for its remarkable arsenal of antioxidants. These microscopic warriors play a crucial role in defending our bodies against the ravages of time and disease, making cacao a true champion of health and longevity.

Understanding Antioxidants: The Body's Defense System

Before we delve into cacao's specific antioxidant power, let's understand what antioxidants are and why they are so important for our health. In essence, antioxidants are molecules that protect our cells from damage caused by free radicals. Free radicals are unstable molecules that are produced naturally in our bodies as a byproduct of metabolism, but they can also be generated by external factors like pollution, smoking, and radiation. When free radicals accumulate, they can cause oxidative stress, a process that damages cells and contributes to aging and various diseases, including cancer, heart disease, and neurodegenerative disorders.

Antioxidants work by neutralizing free radicals, preventing them from causing damage to our cells. They act as scavengers, donating electrons to stabilize free radicals and render them harmless. By protecting our cells from oxidative stress, antioxidants play a crucial role in maintaining overall health and well-being.

Cacao's Antioxidant Powerhouse: A Rich Source of Flavanols and Polyphenols

Cacao is a true antioxidant powerhouse, boasting one of the

highest concentrations of antioxidants found in any food. The primary antioxidants in cacao are flavanols, a type of flavonoid that's been extensively studied for its health benefits. Flavanols have been shown to have powerful antioxidant and anti-inflammatory effects, protecting cells from damage and reducing the risk of chronic diseases.

In addition to flavanols, cacao also contains other types of antioxidants, including proanthocyanidins and catechins. These compounds work synergistically with flavanols to provide a comprehensive defense against oxidative stress. Studies have shown that consuming cacao can significantly increase the level of antioxidants in the bloodstream, providing a protective shield for our cells.

Fighting Disease: Cacao's Potential Role in Prevention

The antioxidant properties of cacao have been linked to a wide range of health benefits, including reduced risk of heart disease, cancer, and neurodegenerative disorders. By neutralizing free radicals and reducing inflammation, cacao may help prevent the development of these chronic diseases.

For example, studies have shown that cacao consumption can improve cholesterol levels, reduce blood pressure, and improve blood vessel function, all of which are important factors in heart health. Cacao has also been shown to inhibit the growth of cancer cells and reduce inflammation, which may play a role in cancer prevention. Additionally, the antioxidant and anti-inflammatory effects of cacao may protect the brain from damage and potentially reduce the risk of neurodegenerative diseases like Alzheimer's and Parkinson's.

The Anti-Aging Elixir: Cacao's Potential for Longevity

The antioxidant properties of cacao have also sparked interest in its potential anti-aging effects. By protecting cells from damage and reducing inflammation, cacao may help slow down the aging process and promote longevity. While more research is needed to fully understand the anti-aging potential of cacao, the existing evidence suggests that it may be a valuable addition to a healthy lifestyle.

Maximizing Cacao's Benefits: Choosing the Right Chocolate

While cacao is a potent source of antioxidants, it's important to note that not all chocolate is created equal. The antioxidant content of chocolate varies depending on the type and processing methods. Dark chocolate with a high percentage of cacao solids (70% or higher) generally contains the highest levels of antioxidants. Milk chocolate and white chocolate, which contain less cacao and more sugar and fat, offer fewer antioxidant benefits.

To maximize the antioxidant benefits of cacao, choose dark chocolate with a high cacao content, and enjoy it in moderation as part of a balanced diet. You can also incorporate raw cacao nibs or cacao powder into your smoothies, desserts, or other recipes for a delicious and nutritious boost of antioxidants.

Cacao's antioxidant arsenal is a testament to its status as a superfood. By protecting our cells from damage and reducing the risk of chronic diseases, cacao offers a delicious and natural way to promote health and longevity. So, indulge in this ancient elixir and savor its rich flavor, knowing that you're also nourishing your body from the inside out.

THE GUT FEELING: CACAO'S ROLE IN DIGESTIVE HEALTH

It's no secret that the foods we eat have a profound impact on our overall well-being. But what you might not know is that cacao, the heart and soul of chocolate, is emerging as a surprising champion for digestive health. Beyond its delectable taste and mood-boosting properties, cacao offers a range of benefits that nourish and support our gut, the foundation of our overall health.

Fiber: Fuel for a Flourishing Microbiome

One of cacao's most significant contributions to digestive health is its rich fiber content. Fiber is a type of carbohydrate that the body cannot digest, but it plays a crucial role in maintaining a healthy gut. It acts as a prebiotic, providing nourishment for the beneficial bacteria that reside in our intestines, collectively known as the gut microbiome. This diverse community of microorganisms plays a vital role in digestion, immune function, and overall health.

Cacao contains both soluble and insoluble fiber. Soluble fiber dissolves in water and forms a gel-like substance that helps slow down digestion and promotes regular bowel movements. Insoluble fiber, on the other hand, adds bulk to the stool and helps move waste through the digestive tract more efficiently. By providing both types of fiber, cacao supports a balanced and healthy gut microbiome, promoting optimal digestion and nutrient absorption.

Polyphenols: Powerful Anti-Inflammatory Agents

Cacao is also rich in polyphenols, plant compounds that have been shown to have anti-inflammatory effects in the gut. Chronic inflammation in the gut can disrupt the delicate balance of the microbiome, leading to digestive problems like irritable bowel syndrome (IBS), inflammatory bowel disease (IBD), and even leaky gut syndrome. The polyphenols in cacao can help reduce inflammation, soothe irritated tissues, and promote the growth of beneficial bacteria, contributing to a healthier and happier gut.

Prebiotic Potential: Nurturing Beneficial Bacteria

In addition to its fiber content, cacao also contains compounds that have prebiotic potential, meaning they can selectively stimulate the growth and activity of beneficial bacteria in the gut. These compounds include oligosaccharides and polyphenols, which act as fuel for specific strains of bacteria that are known to promote digestive health. By nurturing these beneficial bacteria, cacao can help maintain a balanced microbiome, which is crucial for optimal digestion and overall well-being.

Improved Gut Barrier Function: Protecting Against Leaky Gut

Another way cacao supports digestive health is by improving the integrity of the gut barrier. The gut barrier is a semi-permeable lining that separates the contents of the intestines from the rest of the body. When this barrier becomes compromised, a condition known as leaky gut syndrome, harmful substances can leak into the bloodstream, triggering inflammation and potentially contributing to various health problems. Cacao contains compounds that can help strengthen the gut barrier, protecting against leaky gut and promoting optimal digestive function.

A Holistic Approach to Digestive Health: More than Just a Treat

Cacao's benefits for digestive health extend beyond its individual components. The combination of fiber, polyphenols, prebiotics, and other beneficial compounds creates a synergistic effect that promotes a healthy and balanced gut microbiome. By incorporating cacao into your diet, you can nourish your gut from the inside out, supporting optimal digestion, nutrient absorption, and overall well-being.

While enjoying cacao in the form of dark chocolate is a delicious way to reap its digestive benefits, it's important to choose chocolate with a high percentage of cacao solids (70% or higher) and minimal added sugar. You can also incorporate raw cacao nibs or cacao powder into smoothies, desserts, or other recipes for a nutritious and flavorful boost.

As we continue to uncover the secrets of the gut microbiome and its impact on our health, cacao emerges as a promising ally in our quest for optimal digestive health. By nourishing our gut with this ancient superfood, we can unlock a wealth of benefits that extend far beyond the pleasure of indulging in a delicious treat.

THE CHOCOLATE RITUALS: CULTURAL SIGNIFICANCE AND TRADITIONS

The allure of chocolate transcends mere taste and nutrition; it has woven itself into the cultural fabric of societies across the globe, becoming an integral part of rituals, celebrations, and everyday life. From ancient Mesoamerican civilizations to modern-day festivities, chocolate has held a unique and often sacred place in human traditions.

Ancient Reverence: Cacao Ceremonies and Rituals

Long before chocolate became a global commodity, it was a sacred elixir revered by Mesoamerican cultures. The Maya and Aztec civilizations, in particular, held cacao in high esteem, believing it to be a gift from the gods. Cacao beans were used as currency, offered as tribute to rulers, and incorporated into elaborate rituals and ceremonies.

These ancient rituals often involved the preparation and consumption of xocolatl, a bitter, frothy drink made from roasted cacao beans, water, chili peppers, and spices. Xocolatl was not merely a beverage; it was a conduit to the divine, believed to enhance spiritual connection, induce visions, and offer guidance from ancestors. Cacao ceremonies were often accompanied by music, dance, and other forms of artistic expression, creating a multisensory experience that celebrated the sacredness of cacao.

Cacao and Royalty: A Symbol of Power and Prestige

In many ancient cultures, cacao was reserved for the elite, a symbol of power and prestige. Mayan and Aztec rulers consumed xocolatl during important ceremonies and state occasions, believing it enhanced their strength, wisdom, and connection to the divine. Cacao beans were also given as gifts to dignitaries and used to forge alliances between different kingdoms.

The association of cacao with royalty continued in Europe after its introduction by Spanish conquistadors. European monarchs and aristocrats embraced chocolate as a symbol of luxury and refinement, indulging in elaborate chocolate rituals and commissioning exquisite chocolate services crafted from precious metals.

Chocolate and Celebrations: Sweetening Life's Milestones

As chocolate became more accessible to the general population, it found its way into a variety of celebrations and festivities. In many cultures, chocolate is associated with joy, happiness, and love. It is often given as a gift on special occasions like birthdays, anniversaries, and holidays.

Chocolate plays a central role in many cultural traditions. In Mexico, Dia de los Muertos (Day of the Dead) celebrations feature offerings of chocolate to deceased loved ones. In Italy, Easter is marked by the consumption of chocolate eggs, symbolizing new life and fertility. In the United States, Valentine's Day is synonymous with boxes of chocolates, a sweet expression of love and affection.

Chocolate and Everyday Rituals: Comfort and Connection

Beyond special occasions, chocolate has also become integrated into our daily rituals. A morning cup of hot chocolate can provide a comforting start to the day, while a piece of dark chocolate after dinner can offer a satisfying end to a meal. Chocolate is often shared among friends and family, fostering connection and creating moments of shared pleasure.

The Ritual of Chocolate Making: A Modern Tradition

In recent years, there has been a resurgence of interest in the art of chocolate making. Bean-to-bar chocolate makers are reviving traditional techniques and emphasizing the importance of quality ingredients and ethical sourcing. This movement celebrates the craftsmanship and cultural significance of chocolate, connecting consumers with the origins of their favorite treat.

Cacao ceremonies, inspired by ancient practices, are also gaining popularity. These ceremonies create a space for participants to connect with the spiritual and medicinal properties of cacao, fostering mindfulness, creativity, and personal growth.

The cultural significance of chocolate is a testament to its enduring power to bring people together, celebrate life's milestones, and offer comfort and joy. From ancient rituals to modern traditions, chocolate continues to play a central role in our lives, reminding us of the power of food to nourish our bodies, minds, and spirits.

MODERN CHOCOLATE MOVEMENTS: FAIR TRADE, SINGLE ORIGIN, AND BEAN-TO-BAR

The world of chocolate is undergoing a revolution, one that's driven by a growing awareness of social responsibility, a desire for transparency, and a newfound appreciation for the craft of chocolate making. Three movements – Fair Trade, Single Origin, and Bean-to-Bar – are at the forefront of this change, transforming the way we perceive and consume chocolate.

Fair Trade: A Sweet Deal for Farmers and Consumers

Fair Trade is a global movement that aims to create a more equitable and sustainable system for farmers and workers in developing countries. In the context of chocolate, Fair Trade certification ensures that cacao farmers receive a fair price for their beans, protecting them from volatile market fluctuations and enabling them to invest in their communities and livelihoods. Fair Trade standards also prohibit child labor and forced labor, promote safe and healthy working conditions, and encourage environmentally sustainable farming practices.

For consumers, choosing Fair Trade chocolate is a way to support ethical and sustainable practices in the cacao industry. By purchasing Fair Trade certified products, we can help empower farmers, improve their livelihoods, and contribute to a more just and equitable global economy. Fair Trade chocolate is widely available in supermarkets and specialty stores, making it easy for consumers to make a conscious choice.

Single Origin: A Taste of Terroir

Single Origin chocolate is made from cacao beans sourced from a specific region or even a single plantation. This allows the unique flavors and characteristics of the cacao to shine through, much like wine from a particular vineyard. Single Origin chocolate often has a complex flavor profile, reflecting the terroir of the region where the cacao beans were grown. Factors like soil composition, climate, and altitude can all influence the flavor of cacao, resulting in a diverse range of taste experiences.

For chocolate enthusiasts, Single Origin chocolate offers a journey of discovery. Each bar tells a story of its origin, showcasing the unique flavors and nuances of a particular region. It's an opportunity to appreciate the craftsmanship of chocolate making and the diversity of cacao varieties around the world. Single Origin chocolate is becoming increasingly popular, with many craft chocolate makers specializing in this unique category.

Bean-to-Bar: The Craft Chocolate Revolution

The Bean-to-Bar movement is a celebration of craftsmanship and transparency in chocolate making. Bean-to-Bar chocolate makers source their cacao beans directly from farmers, ensuring fair prices and ethical practices. They then control every step of the chocolate-making process, from roasting and grinding the beans to conching and tempering the chocolate. This hands-on approach allows them to create unique flavor profiles and showcase the quality of their ingredients.

Bean-to-Bar chocolate is often made in small batches, using minimal ingredients and avoiding artificial flavors and preservatives. This results in a purer, more authentic chocolate experience that highlights the natural flavors of cacao. Bean-to-Bar chocolate makers are passionate about their craft and often share their knowledge and expertise with consumers, creating a deeper appreciation for the art of chocolate making.

The Impact of Modern Chocolate Movements

The Fair Trade, Single Origin, and Bean-to-Bar movements are transforming the chocolate industry, promoting ethical sourcing, transparency, and craftsmanship. They are empowering farmers, improving livelihoods, and creating a more sustainable and equitable future for cacao. For consumers, these movements offer a wider range of choices and a deeper understanding of the chocolate they consume. By choosing Fair Trade, Single Origin, or Bean-to-Bar chocolate, we can support positive change in the industry and savor the true essence of cacao.

CACAO CEREMONIES: ANCIENT WISDOM FOR MODERN HEALING

In our fast-paced, technology-driven world, finding moments of stillness and connection can be a challenge. Yet, an ancient practice is resurfacing, offering a path to inner peace, healing, and spiritual awakening: the cacao ceremony. Rooted in the traditions of Mesoamerican cultures, cacao ceremonies are experiencing a resurgence in modern times, attracting those seeking a deeper connection to themselves, others, and the natural world.

A Sacred Gathering: Honoring the Spirit of Cacao

Cacao ceremonies are intentional gatherings where participants consume a specially prepared cacao drink in a ceremonial setting. Unlike casual chocolate consumption, cacao ceremonies are infused with reverence and intention, honoring the sacred history and spiritual significance of cacao. The ceremonies often incorporate elements like meditation, music, breathwork, and sharing circles, creating a safe and supportive space for participants to explore their inner landscape and connect with the healing energy of cacao.

The Cacao Elixir: A Heart-Opening Medicine

The cacao used in ceremonies is typically prepared in a traditional manner, using raw, unprocessed cacao beans that have been minimally heated to preserve their nutritional and energetic properties. The beans are ground into a paste and mixed with water and spices like cinnamon, cayenne pepper, and cardamom. This creates a rich, bitter drink that is believed to open the heart, enhance intuition, and promote emotional healing.

Cacao contains a unique combination of compounds that can support physical, mental, and emotional well-being. Theobromine, a mild stimulant, provides a gentle energy boost, while anandamide, the "bliss molecule," promotes relaxation and euphoria. Cacao also contains magnesium, a mineral that supports muscle relaxation and stress reduction.

A Journey of Inner Exploration: The Cacao Experience

Cacao ceremonies are often described as a journey of inner exploration and self-discovery. The ceremonial setting, combined with the unique properties of cacao, can create a heightened state of awareness and receptivity. Participants may experience a range of emotions, from joy and gratitude to sadness and grief. The cacao is believed to facilitate the release of emotional blockages, allowing for deeper healing and transformation.

The ceremonial aspect of cacao consumption also creates a sense of community and connection. Sharing the cacao drink with others in a sacred space fosters a feeling of unity and belonging, allowing participants to feel supported and understood. The ceremonies often include sharing circles, where individuals can express their thoughts, feelings, and experiences in a safe and non-judgmental environment.

Modern Adaptations: Cacao Ceremonies for the 21st Century

While cacao ceremonies are rooted in ancient traditions, they have been adapted to meet the needs of modern seekers. Many facilitators incorporate elements like sound healing, guided meditations, and energy work into their ceremonies, creating a unique and personalized experience for participants.

Cacao ceremonies are becoming increasingly popular as people seek alternative ways to connect with themselves, others, and the natural world. They offer a respite from the demands of modern life, providing a space for reflection, introspection, and healing.

The Science Behind the Ceremony: Cacao's Therapeutic Potential

While cacao ceremonies are often described in spiritual terms, there is also scientific evidence to support the therapeutic potential of cacao. Studies have shown that cacao can improve mood, reduce stress, and enhance cognitive function. The combination of theobromine, anandamide, magnesium, and other compounds in cacao creates a synergistic effect that promotes relaxation, well-being, and emotional balance.

Cacao ceremonies offer a unique way to experience the healing power of cacao in a supportive and intentional setting. Whether you are seeking emotional healing, spiritual connection, or simply a moment of peace and relaxation, cacao ceremonies can provide a transformative experience.

The resurgence of cacao ceremonies is a testament to the enduring wisdom of ancient cultures and the power of cacao to connect us with our inner selves and the world around us. By honoring the sacredness of cacao and embracing its healing potential, we can create a space for personal growth, transformation, and collective well-being.

CHOCOLATE THERAPY: INDULGENCE FOR MIND, BODY, AND SPIRIT

Chocolate, often associated with indulgence and guilty pleasure, is undergoing a paradigm shift. It's no longer just a sweet treat; it's being recognized as a form of therapy that can nourish the mind, body, and spirit. Chocolate therapy is an emerging field that explores the therapeutic potential of chocolate, harnessing its unique properties to promote relaxation, reduce stress, and enhance overall well-being.

The Sensory Experience: A Symphony of Pleasure

Chocolate therapy begins with the sensory experience of indulging in chocolate. The rich aroma, velvety texture, and complex flavors stimulate our senses, creating a moment of pure pleasure. This sensory delight triggers the release of endorphins, our body's natural feel-good chemicals, promoting a sense of happiness and relaxation. The act of savoring chocolate can be a form of mindfulness, allowing us to focus on the present moment and let go of worries and stress.

Mood Enhancement: The Science of Chocolate-Induced Bliss

Beyond the sensory experience, chocolate contains compounds that have been shown to have a positive impact on mood. Theobromine, a mild stimulant, provides a gentle energy boost, while anandamide, the "bliss molecule," promotes relaxation and euphoria. Phenylethylamine (PEA), a neurotransmitter associated with feelings of love and attraction, is also present in chocolate, potentially contributing to its reputation as an aphrodisiac.

Studies have shown that consuming chocolate can increase serotonin levels in the brain, a neurotransmitter that plays a crucial role in regulating mood, sleep, and appetite. Serotonin is often referred to as the "happiness hormone" because it promotes feelings of calmness, contentment, and well-being. By boosting serotonin levels, chocolate can act as a natural mood elevator, helping to alleviate symptoms of depression and anxiety.

Stress Reduction: Cacao's Calming Effect

Chocolate's mood-boosting properties also extend to stress reduction. The flavonoids in cacao have been shown to have a calming effect on the nervous system, reducing the production of stress hormones like cortisol. Additionally, the magnesium in chocolate can help relax muscles and promote a sense of calmness. By reducing stress and promoting relaxation, chocolate can help us cope with the challenges of daily life and improve our overall well-being.

Chocolate and Mindfulness: Savoring the Moment

Mindfulness, the practice of paying attention to the present moment without judgment, is a powerful tool for reducing stress and improving mental health. Chocolate can be incorporated into mindfulness practices, allowing us to fully engage our senses and savor the experience of eating. By focusing on the aroma, texture, and taste of chocolate, we can cultivate a deeper appreciation for this simple pleasure and connect with the present moment.

Chocolate and Self-Care: Indulgence with Intention

Chocolate therapy encourages us to embrace chocolate as a form of self-care, a way to nourish our bodies and minds. It's about indulging in moderation, with intention and awareness. By savoring chocolate mindfully, we can transform it from a guilty pleasure into a source of nourishment and well-being.

Chocolate therapy is not a substitute for professional mental health treatment, but it can be a valuable complementary approach. By incorporating chocolate into our self-care routine, we can harness its mood-boosting, stress-reducing, and mindfulness-enhancing properties to promote overall well-being and create a more joyful and balanced life.

BEYOND THE BAR: CREATIVE CULINARY USES OF CACAO

While chocolate bars are the most common way to enjoy cacao, this versatile ingredient has so much more to offer beyond the confines of a candy wrapper. Cacao's unique flavor profile, nutritional value, and versatility make it a star player in a wide range of culinary creations, from savory dishes to innovative desserts. Let's explore the many ways cacao can be used to elevate your cooking and expand your culinary horizons.

Cacao Nibs: A Crunchy and Nutritious Addition

Cacao nibs, the roasted and crushed bits of cacao beans, are a versatile ingredient that can add a unique texture and flavor to both sweet and savory dishes. Their slightly bitter, chocolatey flavor and crunchy texture make them a great addition to trail mixes, granola bars, and yogurt parfaits. They can also be sprinkled on salads, incorporated into grain bowls, or used as a topping for roasted vegetables, adding a touch of complexity and depth to otherwise simple dishes.

Cacao Powder: A Rich and Versatile Flavor Enhancer

Cacao powder, made from finely ground cacao beans, is a pantry staple for many home cooks and chefs. Its rich, chocolatey flavor can be used to create a wide range of dishes, from decadent desserts to savory sauces and marinades. Cacao powder can be used to make hot chocolate, brownies, cakes, cookies, and other classic chocolate treats. It can also be added to smoothies, protein shakes, and even savory dishes like chili, mole sauce, and barbecue rubs. The possibilities are endless, limited only by your imagination.

Cacao Butter: A Luxurious and Healthy Fat

Cacao butter, the natural fat extracted from cacao beans, is a luxurious ingredient that can elevate your cooking to new heights. Its smooth, creamy texture and subtle chocolatey aroma make it a perfect substitute for butter or oil in baking and cooking. Cacao butter can be used to make dairy-free chocolate, vegan desserts, and even savory dishes like roasted vegetables and risotto. It's also a popular ingredient in skincare products, thanks to its moisturizing and nourishing properties.

Cacao Liquor: The Pure Essence of Chocolate Flavor

Cacao liquor, also known as unsweetened chocolate, is the purest form of chocolate, made by grinding roasted cacao beans into a liquid. It has a deep, intense chocolate flavor and a slightly gritty texture. Cacao liquor is a key ingredient in many chocolate confections, but it can also be used to create unique savory dishes. Try adding it to stews, braises, or even homemade barbecue sauce for a surprising depth of flavor.

Beyond the Kitchen: Cacao in Beverages and Beyond

Cacao's culinary applications extend beyond the kitchen. Cacao beans can be brewed into a rich, flavorful tea that offers a gentle energy boost and a unique taste experience. Cacao can also be used to make alcoholic beverages like chocolate liqueur and cacao-infused beer. And for the adventurous, cacao can even be incorporated into savory cocktails, adding a touch of complexity and intrigue to classic drinks.

Embracing Cacao's Culinary Potential

Cacao is a versatile ingredient that can be used in countless ways to elevate your cooking and expand your culinary repertoire. Whether you're a seasoned chef or a home cook looking to experiment, cacao offers a world of possibilities. By embracing cacao's culinary potential, you can create dishes that are not only delicious but also nutritious and satisfying.

So, the next time you reach for a chocolate bar, consider exploring the many other ways to enjoy this versatile ingredient. From cacao nibs and powder to cacao butter and liquor, cacao offers a wealth of culinary possibilities. By incorporating cacao into your cooking, you can discover new flavors, textures, and experiences that will delight your taste buds and nourish your body.

42

CACAO BEAUTY SECRETS: NOURISHING SKIN AND HAIR

The allure of cacao extends beyond the kitchen and into the realm of beauty. For centuries, cultures around the world have recognized the skin-loving and hair-nourishing properties of cacao, incorporating it into various beauty rituals and remedies. Today, modern science is catching up with ancient wisdom, uncovering the secrets behind cacao's beautifying effects.

Cacao Butter: Nature's Moisturizer

At the heart of cacao's beauty benefits lies cacao butter, a rich, emollient fat extracted from cacao beans. Cacao butter is a natural moisturizer that deeply hydrates and nourishes the skin. It's packed with essential fatty acids, including oleic acid, stearic acid, and palmitic acid, which help to replenish the skin's natural moisture barrier, preventing dryness and dehydration.

Cacao butter is also rich in antioxidants, such as flavanols and polyphenols, which protect the skin from damage caused by free radicals. Free radicals are unstable molecules that can damage skin cells and accelerate the aging process. By neutralizing free radicals, cacao butter helps to maintain the skin's elasticity, firmness, and youthful glow.

Cacao for Glowing Skin: Benefits Beyond Moisturizing

Beyond its moisturizing properties, cacao offers a range of other benefits for the skin. The antioxidants in cacao help to reduce inflammation, soothe irritated skin, and promote healing. Cacao also contains caffeine, which can stimulate blood flow and improve circulation, giving the skin a healthy, radiant glow.

Cacao is also a natural source of vitamins and minerals, including vitamin E, magnesium, and iron. These nutrients are essential for healthy skin, promoting cell regeneration, collagen production, and overall skin health. Vitamin E, in particular, is a powerful antioxidant that protects the skin from damage caused by UV rays and environmental pollutants.

Cacao for Luscious Locks: Nourishing Hair from Root to Tip

The benefits of cacao extend beyond the skin, reaching all the way to the tips of your hair. Cacao butter is a natural conditioner that can help to soften and hydrate dry, damaged hair. It can also help to detangle hair, reduce frizz, and add shine.

Cacao is also a good source of sulfur, a mineral that is essential for healthy hair growth. Sulfur is a component of keratin, the protein that makes up our hair. By providing sulfur, cacao can help to strengthen hair follicles, prevent breakage, and promote healthy hair growth.

Cacao Beauty Rituals: Ancient Wisdom for Modern Times

For centuries, cultures around the world have used cacao in their beauty rituals. In ancient Mesoamerica, cacao was used to create luxurious body masks and hair treatments. Mayan women would mix cacao butter with honey and herbs to create a nourishing mask for their skin, while Aztec warriors would use cacao butter to protect their skin from the sun and elements.

Today, we can incorporate cacao into our own beauty rituals, drawing on the wisdom of ancient cultures. Cacao butter can be used as a natural moisturizer, lip balm, or hair mask. It can also be added to homemade soaps, lotions, and scrubs. Cacao powder can be mixed with honey and yogurt to create a revitalizing face mask.

Incorporating Cacao into Your Beauty Routine

There are many ways to incorporate cacao into your beauty routine. You can use pure cacao butter, cacao powder, or even dark chocolate with a high cacao content. Here are a few simple ideas to get you started:

- **Cacao Butter Moisturizer:** Apply a small amount of cacao butter to your face and body after showering or bathing. It will melt into your skin, leaving it feeling soft, supple, and hydrated.
- **Cacao Lip Balm:** Melt cacao butter and combine it with a few drops of essential oil, such as peppermint or lavender, to create a nourishing and flavorful lip balm.
- **Cacao Hair Mask:** Mix cacao powder with honey, yogurt, and olive oil to create a hydrating and nourishing hair mask. Apply it to your hair, leave it on for 30 minutes, and then rinse thoroughly.
- **Cacao Face Mask:** Combine cacao powder with honey and mashed avocado for a revitalizing face mask that will leave your skin feeling soft and glowing.

By incorporating cacao into your beauty routine, you can harness its nourishing and beautifying properties to achieve healthy, radiant skin and hair. So, go ahead and indulge in the sweet luxury of cacao, not just for its delicious taste but also for its ability to enhance your natural beauty.

THE CACAO ECONOMY: EMPOWERING FARMERS AND COMMUNITIES

The global love affair with chocolate is undeniable, but behind every delicious bar lies a complex economic system that impacts the lives of millions of cacao farmers and their communities. Understanding the cacao economy is essential for appreciating the true cost of chocolate and the potential for this humble bean to transform lives and create a more equitable and sustainable world.

Small-Scale Farmers: The Backbone of the Cacao Industry

Cacao is primarily grown by small-scale farmers in tropical regions around the world, including West Africa, Latin America, and Southeast Asia. These farmers, often living in remote areas with limited access to resources, are the backbone of the cacao industry. Their hard work and dedication bring us the raw material that is transformed into the chocolate we enjoy.

Yet, many cacao farmers face significant challenges. Low prices for their beans, volatile market fluctuations, and lack of access to credit and training can make it difficult for them to earn a decent living and provide for their families. Additionally, climate change, pests, and diseases can threaten their crops and livelihoods.

Fair Trade: A Pathway to Empowerment

One way to address these challenges is through Fair Trade certification. Fair Trade is a global movement that aims to create a more equitable and sustainable system for farmers and workers in developing countries. In the context of cacao, Fair Trade certification ensures that farmers receive a minimum price for their beans, regardless of market fluctuations. This price covers the cost of sustainable production and provides a living wage for farmers and their families.

Fair Trade also promotes community development by requiring that a portion of the price paid for Fair Trade cacao beans goes into a communal fund. This fund is used to support projects that benefit the community, such as education, healthcare, and infrastructure development. Fair Trade certification also prohibits child labor and forced labor, promotes safe and healthy working conditions, and encourages environmentally sustainable farming practices.

By choosing Fair Trade chocolate, consumers can directly support cacao farmers and their communities. This simple act can have a profound impact, empowering farmers to invest in their businesses, send their children to school, and improve their quality of life.

Single Origin and Bean-to-Bar: Creating Value through Quality

Another way to empower cacao farmers is through the Single Origin and Bean-to-Bar movements. Single Origin chocolate highlights the unique flavors and characteristics of cacao beans from a specific region or plantation, often paying a premium price for high-quality beans. This incentivizes farmers to focus on quality and sustainability, rather than simply maximizing yields.

Bean-to-Bar chocolate makers work directly with cacao farmers, building relationships based on trust and mutual respect. They often pay farmers a higher price for their beans and provide training and support to improve farming practices. This direct connection between chocolate makers and farmers creates a sense of ownership and pride, empowering farmers to take control of their livelihoods and build a sustainable future.

Empowering Women in Cacao: A Key to Success

Women play a crucial role in the cacao industry, often responsible for tasks like harvesting, fermenting, and drying the beans.

However, they often face discrimination and have limited access to resources and decision-making power. Empowering women in the cacao industry is not only a matter of gender equality, but it's also a key to improving the livelihoods of farmers and their communities.

Several organizations and initiatives are working to empower women in cacao, providing them with training, access to finance, and leadership opportunities. By supporting these efforts, we can contribute to a more equitable and sustainable cacao industry that benefits everyone involved.

The Future of the Cacao Economy: A Vision for Sustainability and Prosperity

The cacao economy is at a crossroads. The challenges of climate change, pests, diseases, and market volatility threaten the livelihoods of millions of cacao farmers. However, there is also a growing movement towards sustainability, ethical sourcing, and empowerment. By supporting Fair Trade, Single Origin, and Bean-to-Bar chocolate, we can create a demand for high-quality, ethically sourced cacao that benefits farmers, communities, and the environment.

The future of the cacao economy depends on our choices as consumers. By choosing chocolate that is produced in a way that respects people and the planet, we can contribute to a more equitable and sustainable world. It's a small but powerful way to make a difference, one delicious bite at a time.

REGENERATIVE CACAO: CULTIVATING A SUSTAINABLE FUTURE

As the world grapples with the urgent need for sustainable solutions, the cacao industry is undergoing a profound transformation. Regenerative cacao, a holistic approach to farming that focuses on restoring and revitalizing ecosystems, is emerging as a beacon of hope for a more sustainable and equitable future for both people and the planet.

Regenerative Agriculture: A Paradigm Shift in Farming

Regenerative agriculture is a farming philosophy and practice that goes beyond sustainability, aiming to actively improve the health of the soil, biodiversity, and overall ecosystem. It emphasizes building soil fertility, sequestering carbon, conserving water, and promoting biodiversity. Unlike conventional farming methods that often deplete natural resources and contribute to environmental degradation, regenerative agriculture seeks to work in harmony with nature, creating a mutually beneficial relationship between farmers, the land, and the communities they serve.

In the context of cacao, regenerative practices involve a range of techniques aimed at restoring degraded ecosystems, promoting soil health, and increasing biodiversity. This includes agroforestry systems that combine cacao trees with other crops and shade trees, creating a diverse and resilient ecosystem that mimics the natural habitat of cacao. Regenerative farmers also use cover crops to protect the soil from erosion, organic fertilizers to nourish the soil, and natural pest control methods to minimize the use of harmful chemicals.

Environmental Benefits: A Win-Win for People and Planet

The environmental benefits of regenerative cacao are significant. By sequestering carbon in the soil, regenerative cacao farms can help mitigate climate change. Healthy soils also retain more water, reducing the need for irrigation and improving drought resilience. Increased biodiversity on regenerative farms provides habitat for pollinators and other beneficial organisms, creating a more resilient ecosystem that is less susceptible to pests and diseases.

Regenerative cacao also offers social and economic benefits. By improving soil health and productivity, it can increase yields and income for farmers. Additionally, regenerative practices often involve the use of local resources and knowledge, creating jobs and strengthening local economies. Regenerative cacao farms can also become hubs for education and research, promoting knowledge sharing and innovation in the cacao industry.

Empowering Farmers: A Pathway to Resilience and Prosperity

Regenerative cacao is not just about environmental sustainability; it's also about empowering farmers and building resilient communities. By adopting regenerative practices, farmers can reduce their dependence on expensive inputs like chemical fertilizers and pesticides, improving their profitability and reducing their vulnerability to market fluctuations. Regenerative cacao farms also tend to be more resilient to climate change, as healthy soils and diverse ecosystems are better able to withstand extreme weather events.

Furthermore, regenerative cacao can foster a sense of pride and ownership among farmers, as they become stewards of the land and actively participate in the restoration of their ecosystems. This can lead to increased motivation and innovation, as farmers experiment with new techniques and share their knowledge with others.

The Future of Cacao: Regenerative Agriculture as a Catalyst for Change

The regenerative cacao movement is still in its early stages, but it has the potential to transform the cacao industry and create a more sustainable and equitable future for all. By supporting regenerative cacao farmers and choosing chocolate made with regenerative cacao, consumers can play a crucial role in driving this change.

Several organizations and initiatives are working to promote regenerative cacao, providing training, resources, and market access to farmers. These efforts are helping to create a new paradigm for cacao production, one that prioritizes environmental health, social equity, and economic resilience.

As we face the challenges of climate change, biodiversity loss, and social inequality, regenerative cacao offers a glimmer of hope. By cultivating a deeper connection to the land, empowering farmers, and promoting sustainable practices, we can create a cacao industry that nourishes both people and the planet.

CACAO ACTIVISM: THE FIGHT FOR ETHICAL AND SUSTAINABLE CHOCOLATE

The chocolate industry is at a crossroads. While consumers enjoy the sweet indulgence of chocolate, a growing awareness of the social and environmental injustices within the industry is fueling a powerful movement for change. Cacao activism, driven by passionate individuals, organizations, and communities, is fighting for a future where chocolate is not only delicious but also ethical and sustainable.

Unearthing the Bitter Truth: The Dark Side of Chocolate

For decades, the chocolate industry has been plagued by issues such as child labor, forced labor, poverty among farmers, deforestation, and unsustainable farming practices. The majority of cacao is produced in West Africa, where an estimated two million children work in hazardous conditions on cacao farms. These children are often exposed to dangerous tools, pesticides, and long hours of labor, robbing them of their childhood and education.

Additionally, many cacao farmers struggle to make a living wage due to low prices for their beans and volatile market fluctuations. This poverty forces farmers to cut corners, leading to unsustainable farming practices that degrade the environment and perpetuate a cycle of poverty. Deforestation for cacao production is a major contributor to climate change and biodiversity loss, further exacerbating the challenges faced by farmers and their communities.

The Rise of Cacao Activism: A Voice for Change

Cacao activism is a diverse and growing movement that

encompasses a wide range of stakeholders, from farmers and workers to consumers, NGOs, and ethical chocolate companies. Activists are raising awareness of the social and environmental injustices within the chocolate industry, advocating for fair trade practices, sustainable farming methods, and living wages for farmers. They are also promoting transparency and traceability in the supply chain, empowering consumers to make informed choices about the chocolate they purchase.

Cacao activists are working on multiple fronts to achieve their goals. They are lobbying governments to enact stricter regulations on child labor and forced labor. They are partnering with farmers to implement sustainable farming practices and improve their livelihoods. They are educating consumers about the importance of ethical sourcing and fair trade. And they are supporting ethical chocolate companies that are committed to social and environmental responsibility.

Consumer Power: Voting with Your Wallet

One of the most powerful tools of cacao activism is consumer power. By choosing to buy chocolate from ethical brands that prioritize fair trade, sustainability, and transparency, consumers can send a strong message to the industry. They can demand that companies take responsibility for their supply chains and invest in the well-being of farmers and their communities.

The Fairtrade movement has been instrumental in raising awareness of the importance of ethical sourcing and empowering farmers. Fairtrade certification ensures that farmers receive a fair price for their beans and that their communities benefit from social and environmental projects. By choosing Fair Trade chocolate, consumers can directly support these efforts and contribute to a more just and sustainable cacao industry.

Beyond Fair Trade: The Rise of Transparency and Traceability

While Fairtrade certification is an important step, cacao activism is increasingly focusing on the need for greater transparency and traceability in the chocolate supply chain. Consumers want to know where their chocolate comes from, who grew the beans, and under what conditions. They want to be assured that their chocolate is not contributing to child labor, deforestation, or other social and environmental harms.

Some chocolate companies are responding to this demand by implementing blockchain technology to track the journey of cacao beans from farm to factory. This allows consumers to trace the origins of their chocolate and ensure that it meets ethical and sustainable standards. Other companies are investing in direct trade relationships with farmers, building trust and transparency throughout the supply chain.

Challenges and Opportunities: The Path to a Sustainable Future

The fight for ethical and sustainable chocolate is not without its challenges. The chocolate industry is complex and fragmented, with many actors and interests involved. Changing deeply entrenched practices and attitudes requires a sustained effort from all stakeholders. However, there is also a growing recognition that the status quo is unsustainable and that a new model is needed.

The cacao activism movement is a powerful force for change, driven by passion, commitment, and a vision for a more just and sustainable future. By working together, we can transform the chocolate industry into a force for good, one that nourishes both people and the planet.

THE CHOCOLATE CONNOISSEUR: TASTING NOTES AND TERROIR

In a world overflowing with mass-produced chocolate bars, a new breed of chocolate lover is emerging – the chocolate connoisseur. Like wine enthusiasts who discern subtle notes of oak and berries, these discerning palates seek out the unique flavors and nuances that distinguish one chocolate from another. They embark on a sensory journey, exploring the world of cacao through tasting notes and the concept of terroir.

Tasting Chocolate Like a Pro: Beyond Sweet and Bitter

For the uninitiated, chocolate might seem like a simple pleasure, a binary experience of sweet and bitter. But for the chocolate connoisseur, each bite is a complex symphony of flavors, aromas, and textures. Just like wine, coffee, or cheese, chocolate can be analyzed and appreciated on a deeper level, revealing a world of subtle nuances and unexpected delights.

When tasting chocolate, connoisseurs pay attention to a variety of factors. The aroma, or nose, is the first clue, offering hints of fruits, spices, nuts, or even floral notes. The initial taste, or attack, is the first impression on the palate, revealing the dominant flavors. The mid-palate is where the complexity of the chocolate unfolds, with flavors evolving and intertwining. The finish is the lingering taste that remains after the chocolate has melted away, leaving a lasting impression.

Texture also plays a crucial role in the chocolate tasting experience. Is it smooth and creamy, or does it have a gritty texture? Does it melt quickly in the mouth, or does it linger, coating the tongue with flavor? These nuances can reveal much about the quality of the chocolate and the skill of the chocolate maker.

Terroir: The Taste of Place

One of the most fascinating aspects of chocolate tasting is the concept of terroir. Terroir, a French term originally used to describe the influence of soil, climate, and other environmental factors on wine grapes, is now being applied to cacao. Just like wine, the flavor of chocolate is influenced by the terroir of the region where the cacao beans were grown.

Cacao beans grown in different regions have distinct flavor profiles, reflecting the unique characteristics of their environment. For example, cacao from Madagascar might have fruity notes of citrus and berries, while cacao from Venezuela might have earthy notes of nuts and tobacco. Even cacao grown on different plantations within the same region can have subtle differences in flavor, depending on the specific microclimate and soil conditions.

Exploring the World of Cacao: A Sensory Adventure

For chocolate connoisseurs, exploring the world of cacao through tasting notes and terroir is a thrilling adventure. It's an opportunity to discover new flavors, appreciate the diversity of cacao varieties, and deepen their understanding of the chocolate-making process.

Chocolate tastings are becoming increasingly popular, offering a guided experience for those who want to learn more about the nuances of chocolate. These tastings often feature a variety of chocolate bars from different origins, allowing participants to compare and contrast flavors, aromas, and textures.

In addition to tastings, chocolate connoisseurs can also deepen their knowledge through books, articles, and online resources. There are numerous guides and resources available that delve into the intricacies of chocolate tasting, providing detailed information on different cacao varieties, flavor profiles, and tasting techniques.

The Rise of Craft Chocolate: A Celebration of Flavor and Origin

The growing interest in chocolate tasting and terroir has fueled the rise of craft chocolate, a movement that emphasizes quality, transparency, and a deep respect for the origins of cacao. Craft chocolate makers source their cacao beans directly from farmers, often paying a premium price for high-quality beans. They then carefully roast and process the beans to create chocolate that showcases the unique flavors of each origin.

Craft chocolate is often made in small batches, using minimal ingredients and avoiding artificial flavors and preservatives. This results in a purer, more authentic chocolate experience that highlights the natural flavors of cacao. Craft chocolate makers are passionate about their craft and often share their knowledge and expertise with consumers, creating a deeper appreciation for the art of chocolate making.

The chocolate connoisseur movement is a celebration of flavor, origin, and craftsmanship. It's a reminder that chocolate is more than just a sweet treat; it's a complex and nuanced culinary experience that can be appreciated on a deeper level. By exploring the world of cacao through tasting notes and terroir, we can expand our palates, discover new flavors, and deepen our appreciation for this extraordinary bean.

THE FUTURE OF CACAO: EMERGING TRENDS AND INNOVATIONS

The world of cacao is constantly evolving, with exciting trends and innovations shaping the future of this beloved superfood. From groundbreaking scientific discoveries to creative culinary applications and sustainable farming practices, the cacao revolution is far from over. Let's delve into the emerging trends that are poised to transform the way we perceive, consume, and appreciate cacao.

Health and Wellness: Cacao's Rising Star

Cacao's health benefits are no longer a secret. As scientific research continues to uncover the numerous ways in which cacao can enhance our well-being, it's no surprise that it's becoming a star ingredient in the health and wellness industry.

Functional Chocolate: A Delicious Dose of Wellness

Functional chocolate, infused with additional health-boosting ingredients like probiotics, adaptogens, or superfoods, is gaining popularity. This trend reflects a growing demand for products that offer both pleasure and nourishment. Whether it's chocolate enriched with gut-friendly probiotics or a bar infused with stress-relieving adaptogens, functional chocolate is a delicious way to incorporate cacao's health benefits into your daily routine.

Personalized Nutrition: Cacao for Your Unique Needs

The rise of personalized nutrition is also impacting the cacao industry. With advancements in genetic testing and microbiome analysis, consumers are seeking personalized recommendations for their diet and lifestyle. Cacao, with its diverse range of nutrients and bioactive compounds, can be tailored to individual needs. For example, someone with high blood pressure may benefit from flavanol-rich dark chocolate, while someone looking to boost their mood may opt for a chocolate bar with added tryptophan.

Cacao and Gut Health: A Blossoming Relationship

The gut microbiome, a complex community of microorganisms residing in our digestive tract, is emerging as a key player in our overall health. Research suggests that a healthy gut microbiome is essential for digestion, immune function, mental health, and even weight management. Cacao, with its prebiotic fiber and polyphenols, has been shown to promote a healthy gut microbiome. As our understanding of the gut-brain connection deepens, we can expect to see more innovative cacao products targeting gut health, such as probiotic-infused chocolate or cacao supplements designed to nourish the microbiome.

Sustainability and Ethics: The Future of Cacao Farming

As consumers become more conscious of the environmental and social impact of their food choices, the cacao industry is responding with a renewed focus on sustainability and ethics.

Regenerative Cacao: A New Paradigm for Farming

Regenerative agriculture, a holistic approach to farming that focuses on restoring and revitalizing ecosystems, is gaining momentum in the cacao industry. Regenerative cacao farms prioritize soil health, biodiversity, and carbon sequestration, creating a more sustainable and resilient system for both farmers and the environment. By choosing chocolate made with regenerative cacao, consumers can support these practices and contribute to a more positive impact on the planet.

Blockchain Technology: Ensuring Transparency and Traceability

Blockchain technology, a decentralized digital ledger that records transactions in a secure and transparent way, is being used to track the journey of cacao beans from farm to factory. This allows consumers to trace the origins of their chocolate and ensure that it meets ethical and sustainable standards. Blockchain can also empower farmers by providing them with a digital identity and a secure way to receive payments, reducing the risk of exploitation and ensuring fair compensation for their labor.

Beyond the Bar: Cacao's Culinary Renaissance

The culinary world is also embracing cacao's versatility, with chefs and food innovators exploring new and exciting ways to incorporate this ingredient into their creations.

Cacao in Savory Cuisine: A Flavorful Twist

Cacao is no longer confined to the dessert menu. Chefs are experimenting with cacao in savory dishes, adding depth and complexity to sauces, marinades, and even main courses. Cacao nibs can be used to add a crunchy texture and a hint of bitterness to salads and grain bowls, while cacao powder can be used to create unique spice rubs for meats and vegetables. Cacao liquor, the pure, unsweetened form of chocolate, is finding its way into stews, braises, and even cocktails, adding a layer of rich, umami flavor.

Cacao-Infused Beverages: More Than Just Hot Chocolate

While hot chocolate remains a beloved classic, cacao is also making a splash in the beverage world in other forms. Cacao tea, brewed from cacao bean husks, is a caffeine-free alternative to coffee that offers a unique flavor profile and a range of health benefits. Cacao is also being used to create innovative alcoholic beverages, such as cacao-infused beer, wine, and even spirits.

The Future of Cacao: A World of Possibilities

The future of cacao is bright, filled with possibilities that extend far beyond the traditional chocolate bar. As we continue to explore the health benefits, culinary versatility, and sustainable potential of cacao, we can expect to see this superfood take center stage in our lives in new and exciting ways. The cacao revolution is here to stay, and it's changing the way we think about, consume, and appreciate this ancient gift from nature.

CACAO FOR KIDS: NURTURING THE NEXT GENERATION OF CHOCOLATE LOVERS

The love for chocolate often begins in childhood, with the first taste of a sweet, milky treat sparking a lifelong passion. But cacao, the raw ingredient in chocolate, offers more than just a sugary delight for kids. It's a nutritional powerhouse packed with essential nutrients and health benefits that can support their growth, development, and overall well-being.

Nutrients for Growing Bodies: Cacao's Nutritional Profile

Cacao is a rich source of essential nutrients that are vital for children's growth and development. It contains magnesium, a mineral that supports bone health, muscle function, and energy production. Cacao is also a good source of iron, which is essential for carrying oxygen throughout the body and preventing anemia. Additionally, cacao contains fiber, which promotes healthy digestion and regularity.

Beyond the Basics: Cacao's Unique Benefits for Kids

In addition to essential nutrients, cacao offers a range of unique benefits that can specifically support children's health and development.

Brain Power: Cacao's Cognitive Boost for Kids

The flavanols in cacao have been shown to improve blood flow to the brain, enhancing cognitive function and focus. Studies have found that children who consume flavanol-rich cocoa beverages show improvements in memory, attention, and problem-solving skills. This cognitive boost can be particularly beneficial for children in school, helping them to learn and concentrate more effectively.

Mood Enhancement: Cacao's Happy Effect on Kids

Cacao's mood-boosting properties can also benefit children. Theobromine, a mild stimulant, provides a gentle energy boost, while anandamide, the "bliss molecule," promotes relaxation and happiness. These compounds, along with other mood-enhancing nutrients like magnesium and tryptophan, can help children feel more positive, balanced, and resilient in the face of stress and challenges.

Immune Support: Cacao's Antioxidant Power for Kids

Cacao's rich antioxidant content can help strengthen children's immune systems and protect them from illness. Antioxidants neutralize harmful free radicals, which can damage cells and contribute to disease. By boosting antioxidant levels in the body, cacao can help support a healthy immune response and reduce the risk of infections.

Energy and Vitality: Cacao's Natural Fuel for Active Kids

Cacao is a natural source of energy, providing a sustained boost without the jitters or crash associated with sugary snacks. Theobromine, a mild stimulant, provides a gentle energy lift, while the natural sugars in cacao provide a quick source of fuel for active kids. Additionally, cacao contains iron, which is essential for carrying oxygen throughout the body and preventing fatigue.

Introducing Cacao to Kids: Fun and Healthy Ways

There are many fun and healthy ways to introduce cacao to children. Here are a few ideas:

- **Smoothies:** Blend cacao powder or nibs into smoothies with fruits, yogurt, and milk for a delicious and nutritious breakfast or snack.
- **Homemade Treats:** Make healthy chocolate treats at home using cacao powder, natural sweeteners like honey or maple syrup, and healthy fats like coconut oil or avocado.

- **Hot Chocolate:** Prepare a warm cup of hot chocolate using cacao powder, milk, and a touch of natural sweetener. This comforting drink is a great way to warm up on a cold day.
- **Cacao Nibs:** Sprinkle cacao nibs on yogurt, oatmeal, or cereal for a crunchy and nutritious topping.

Choosing the Right Chocolate for Kids: Quality and Moderation

When choosing chocolate for kids, it's important to prioritize quality and moderation. Opt for dark chocolate with a high percentage of cacao solids (70% or higher) and minimal added sugar. Dark chocolate offers the most health benefits, while milk chocolate and white chocolate contain less cacao and more sugar. It's also important to limit portion sizes and encourage children to enjoy chocolate as part of a balanced diet.

Cacao: A Delicious Investment in Your Child's Future

By incorporating cacao into your child's diet, you're not just giving them a tasty treat – you're also investing in their health, development, and overall well-being. Cacao's unique combination of nutrients and bioactive compounds can support their growth, enhance their cognitive function, boost their mood, strengthen their immune system, and provide them with natural energy. So, go ahead and share the joy of cacao with your children, knowing that you're giving them a gift that will nourish their bodies and minds for years to come.

CACAO RECIPES: DELICIOUS AND NUTRITIOUS WAYS TO ENJOY THIS SUPERFOOD

Cacao, the magical bean behind our beloved chocolate, is far more versatile than you might think. While indulging in a bar of dark chocolate is a delightful experience, there are countless other ways to enjoy this superfood's rich flavor and reap its remarkable health benefits. In this chapter, we embark on a culinary adventure, exploring delicious and nutritious recipes that showcase the versatility of cacao in both sweet and savory dishes.

Breakfast Delights: Energize Your Day with Cacao

1. Cacao Smoothie Bowl: Start your day with a vibrant and energizing cacao smoothie bowl. Blend frozen bananas, berries, almond milk, and a spoonful of cacao powder until smooth. Top with fresh fruit, granola, and a drizzle of honey for a satisfying and nutritious breakfast that will keep you feeling full and focused.

2. Cacao Overnight Oats: Prepare a jar of overnight oats with rolled oats, chia seeds, milk of choice, and a generous scoop of cacao powder. In the morning, top with your favorite fruits, nuts, and seeds for a grab-and-go breakfast that's packed with protein, fiber, and antioxidants.

Savory Sensations: Cacao Beyond Dessert

3. Mole Sauce: Embark on a culinary adventure with mole sauce, a complex and flavorful Mexican sauce made with cacao, chili peppers, spices, and other ingredients. This rich and savory sauce is traditionally served with chicken or turkey, but it can also be used to elevate

vegetables, tofu, or other proteins.

4. Cacao-Rubbed Steak: Take your steak game to the next level with a cacao-based rub. Combine cacao powder, chili powder, cumin, coriander, salt, and pepper for a smoky, flavorful rub that will add depth and complexity to your grilled or pan-seared steak.

5. Cacao Hummus: Surprise your taste buds with a unique twist on classic hummus. Blend chickpeas, tahini, lemon juice, garlic, olive oil, and a spoonful of cacao powder for a creamy, flavorful dip that's perfect for vegetables, crackers, or pita bread.

Decadent Desserts: Satisfy Your Sweet Tooth with Cacao

6. Flourless Chocolate Cake: Indulge in a rich and decadent flourless chocolate cake made with cacao powder, eggs, butter, and sugar. This gluten-free dessert is surprisingly easy to make and is sure to satisfy even the most discerning chocolate lover.

7. Chocolate Avocado Mousse: This healthy and creamy dessert is a guilt-free indulgence. Blend avocado, cacao powder, maple syrup, and a pinch of salt until smooth. Top with fresh berries and a sprinkle of cacao nibs for a satisfying and nutritious treat.

8. Chocolate Bark: Create a simple yet elegant dessert with chocolate bark. Melt dark chocolate with a high percentage of cacao solids, then spread it onto a parchment-lined baking sheet. Sprinkle with your favorite toppings, such as nuts, seeds, dried fruit, or sea salt, and let it cool and harden. Break into pieces and enjoy.

9. Cacao Truffles: These bite-sized treats are a luxurious indulgence. Combine cacao powder, coconut oil, maple syrup, and a pinch of salt to create a rich and creamy truffle filling. Roll into balls and coat with cacao powder, shredded coconut, or chopped nuts for an elegant and satisfying dessert.

10. Cacao Energy Balls: Fuel your body with these nutritious and delicious energy balls. Combine cacao powder, dates, nut butter, oats, and a pinch of salt in a food processor until a sticky dough forms. Roll into balls and coat with cacao powder or shredded coconut. These energy balls are a perfect snack for a quick energy boost.

Cacao: A Versatile Ingredient for Every Occasion

As you can see, cacao is a versatile ingredient that can be used in a wide range of culinary creations. From breakfast delights to savory sensations and decadent desserts, cacao offers a world of flavor possibilities. By experimenting with different recipes and incorporating cacao into your everyday cooking, you can discover new and exciting ways to enjoy this superfood and reap its numerous health benefits. So, go ahead and unleash your creativity in the kitchen with cacao, and savor the delicious and nutritious results.

CACAO RESOURCES: FURTHER READING, ORGANIZATIONS, AND EXPERTS

The world of cacao is vast and ever-evolving, with a wealth of information, resources, and passionate individuals dedicated to exploring its history, health benefits, culinary potential, and sustainable future. Whether you're a curious newcomer or a seasoned cacao enthusiast, delving deeper into this fascinating world can be a rewarding journey of discovery. This chapter serves as a guide, connecting you with valuable resources, organizations, and experts that can further enrich your cacao knowledge and experience.

Books: Delving Deeper into Cacao's Rich History and Culture

1. The True History of Chocolate by Sophie D. Coe and Michael D. Coe: This comprehensive book explores the fascinating history of cacao, from its ancient origins in Mesoamerica to its global spread and modern-day significance. It delves into the cultural, social, and economic aspects of cacao, offering a rich and nuanced understanding of this beloved bean.

2. Chocolate: A Bittersweet Saga of Dark and Light by Mort Rosenblum: This captivating book takes readers on a journey through the world of chocolate, exploring its history, production, and cultural significance. It delves into the dark side of the chocolate industry, addressing issues like child labor and deforestation, while also celebrating the passion and artistry of chocolate makers.

3. Naked Chocolate: The Astonishing Truth About the World's Greatest Food by David Wolfe and Shazzie:

This informative book explores the health benefits of cacao, highlighting its nutritional value and potential therapeutic properties. It also provides practical tips on how to choose and consume chocolate for optimal health and well-being.

Organizations: Supporting Ethical and Sustainable Cacao

1. Fairtrade International: This global organization promotes fair trade practices in the cacao industry, ensuring that farmers receive a fair price for their beans and that their communities benefit from social and environmental projects. By choosing Fairtrade certified chocolate, you can support ethical sourcing and contribute to a more equitable and sustainable cacao industry.

2. Rainforest Alliance: This international non-profit organization works to conserve biodiversity and ensure sustainable livelihoods by transforming land-use practices, business practices, and consumer behavior. In the cacao industry, the Rainforest Alliance certifies farms that meet rigorous environmental and social standards, promoting sustainable cacao production and protecting rainforests.

3. The Fine Chocolate Industry Association (FCIA): This organization is dedicated to supporting and promoting fine chocolate, which is defined by its high quality, ethical sourcing, and transparency. The FCIA provides resources and education for chocolate makers, retailers, and consumers, fostering a deeper appreciation for the craft of chocolate making and the unique flavors of cacao.

Experts: Learning from the Cacao Masters

1. Maricel Presilla: A renowned chef, culinary historian, and author, Maricel Presilla is a leading authority on the history and culture of cacao and chocolate. Her books, including "The New Taste of Chocolate: A Cultural and Natural History of Cacao with Recipes," offer a wealth of information on cacao's origins, culinary uses, and cultural significance.

2. Mark Sisson: A former elite endurance athlete and bestselling author, Mark Sisson is a proponent of a low-carb, high-fat (ketogenic) diet and lifestyle. He has written extensively about the health benefits of cacao, highlighting its potential to improve cognitive function, boost mood, and support overall health.

3. Clay Gordon: A chocolate educator, consultant, and author, Clay Gordon is a passionate advocate for fine chocolate. He has founded several organizations dedicated to promoting fine chocolate and educating consumers about the importance of quality, ethical sourcing, and transparency.

Online Resources: Expanding Your Cacao Knowledge

1. The Chocolate Life: This online magazine is a treasure trove of information on all things chocolate, from reviews and recipes to news and industry insights. It features articles by experts, interviews with chocolate makers, and a vibrant community forum where chocolate lovers can connect and share their passion.

2. Cacao Magazine: This online publication is dedicated to exploring the world of cacao, covering topics like history, culture, health benefits, and culinary

applications. It features articles by experts, interviews with farmers and chocolate makers, and stunning photography that captures the beauty and diversity of cacao.

3. The Ultimate Chocolate Blog: This blog is a go-to resource for chocolate lovers, offering reviews, recipes, and news from the world of chocolate. It features a wide range of content, from beginner-friendly guides to in-depth explorations of specific cacao origins and chocolate-making techniques.

By exploring these resources, connecting with organizations, and learning from experts, you can deepen your understanding and appreciation for cacao. Whether you're interested in its history, health benefits, culinary uses, or sustainable future, there's a wealth of information waiting to be discovered. So, go forth and explore the captivating world of cacao, and let your passion for this extraordinary bean flourish.

THE CACAO CHALLENGE: 30 DAYS TO TRANSFORM YOUR HEALTH AND HAPPINESS

Are you ready to embark on a delicious journey of transformation? The Cacao Challenge is a 30-day program designed to harness the incredible power of cacao to improve your health, boost your mood, and enhance your overall well-being. It's not a diet or a deprivation plan; it's a celebration of cacao's remarkable benefits and a commitment to nourishing your body and mind with this ancient superfood.

The Power of 30 Days: Creating Lasting Change

Research suggests that it takes about 30 days to form a new habit. The Cacao Challenge is structured to help you create a sustainable cacao routine that you can continue long after the 30 days are over. By incorporating cacao into your daily life in a mindful and intentional way, you can experience lasting changes in your health and happiness.

The Challenge: Embrace Cacao's Magic

The Cacao Challenge is simple yet powerful. For 30 days, you commit to incorporating cacao into your daily routine in various forms. This can include:

- Enjoying a daily cup of cacao tea or hot chocolate made with cacao powder.
- Adding cacao nibs to your smoothies, yogurt, or oatmeal.
- Snacking on dark chocolate with a high percentage of cacao solids.
- Experimenting with cacao recipes in your cooking and baking.
- Participating in a cacao ceremony or meditation.

The key is to choose forms of cacao that are minimally processed and free of added sugar, dairy, or other fillers. Opt for raw cacao powder, cacao nibs, or dark chocolate with a high cacao content to maximize the health benefits.

The Benefits: A Transformation Awaits

By embracing the Cacao Challenge, you can expect to experience a range of benefits for your body, mind, and spirit.

Physical Health:

- Improved heart health: Cacao's flavanols have been shown to lower blood pressure, improve blood vessel function, and reduce the risk of heart disease.
- Enhanced brain function: Cacao's flavanols and other nutrients can improve cognitive function, memory, and focus.
- Boosted immune system: Cacao's antioxidants can strengthen your immune system and protect you from illness.
- Increased energy and vitality: Cacao's natural stimulants and nutrients can provide a sustained energy boost without the jitters or crash.

Mental and Emotional Well-being:

- Reduced stress and anxiety: Cacao's magnesium and other calming compounds can help to reduce stress and promote relaxation.
- Improved mood and happiness: Cacao's mood-boosting compounds like theobromine, anandamide, and phenylethylamine can enhance your mood and create a sense of well-being.
- Increased mindfulness and self-awareness: The act of savoring cacao can be a form of mindfulness, helping you to focus on the present moment and connect with your body and senses.

Beyond the 30 Days: Creating a Cacao-Infused Lifestyle

The Cacao Challenge is just the beginning of your journey with cacao. Once you've completed the 30 days, you can continue to incorporate cacao into your life in a way that feels sustainable and enjoyable. Experiment with different recipes, explore new cacao products, and find ways to make cacao a regular part of your healthy lifestyle.

Remember, the Cacao Challenge is not about perfection; it's about progress. Some days you may indulge in a decadent chocolate dessert, while other days you may simply enjoy a cup of cacao tea. The key is to be mindful of your choices and to focus on the positive impact that cacao can have on your health and happiness.

By embracing the Cacao Challenge, you're not just transforming your diet; you're embarking on a journey of self-discovery and well-being. You're opening yourself up to the magic of cacao, a superfood that has the power to nourish your body, mind, and spirit. So, let's raise a cup of cacao and toast to a healthier, happier you!

THE CACAO MANIFESTO: EMBRACING A CHOCOLATE-FILLED LIFE

We have journeyed together through the rich history, science, culture, and culinary delights of cacao. We have explored its ancient origins, its transformative power on health and well-being, and its potential to create a more sustainable and equitable world. Now, it's time to embrace all that cacao has to offer and incorporate it into our lives in a meaningful and joyful way.

A Manifesto for Cacao Lovers: A Call to Action

This is not just a chapter; it's a manifesto, a call to action for all who cherish the extraordinary gifts of cacao. It's an invitation to embrace a chocolate-filled life, one that celebrates the richness, complexity, and joy that cacao brings to our world.

1. Savor the Experience: Make Chocolate a Mindful Ritual

Chocolate is not merely a snack; it's an experience to be savored. Slow down, engage your senses, and truly appreciate the aroma, texture, and flavor of each bite. Let the act of eating chocolate become a mindful ritual, a moment of pause and pleasure in your busy day.

2. Choose Quality: Opt for Ethical and Sustainable Chocolate

The choices you make as a consumer have a ripple effect on the cacao industry and the planet. Choose chocolate that is ethically sourced, Fair Trade certified, and made with high-quality ingredients. Support brands that prioritize sustainability, transparency, and the well-being of farmers and their communities.

3. Explore the Diversity: Discover the World of Cacao Flavors

Cacao is not a one-size-fits-all ingredient. It comes in a vast array of flavors, aromas, and textures, each reflecting the unique terroir of its origin. Embark on a flavor adventure and explore the world of single-origin chocolate. Discover the fruity notes of Madagascar cacao, the earthy tones of Venezuelan cacao, or the floral hints of Peruvian cacao. Let your taste buds guide you on a journey of discovery.

4. Get Creative in the Kitchen: Experiment with Cacao Recipes

Don't limit yourself to chocolate bars. Cacao can be used in countless ways to elevate your cooking and baking. Experiment with cacao nibs, powder, butter, and liquor to create delicious and nutritious dishes. Try adding cacao to your smoothies, oatmeal, or yogurt for a healthy breakfast boost. Use it to make decadent desserts, savory sauces, or even unique spice rubs for meats and vegetables. Let your culinary creativity soar.

5. Connect with the Cacao Community: Share Your Passion

The cacao community is a vibrant and welcoming space filled with passionate individuals who share a love for this extraordinary bean. Connect with other cacao enthusiasts online or in person, attend chocolate tastings and workshops, and share your discoveries and experiences. By engaging with the community, you can deepen your knowledge, expand your palate, and forge meaningful connections with fellow chocolate lovers.

6. Give Back: Support Organizations That Empower Cacao Farmers

The cacao industry is facing numerous challenges, from poverty and inequality to climate change and deforestation. By supporting organizations that empower cacao farmers and promote sustainable practices, you can contribute to a more equitable and resilient future for the industry. Donate to charities, volunteer your time, or simply spread the word about the importance of ethical and sustainable chocolate.

7. Embrace the Cacao Lifestyle: Nourish Your Body and Mind

Cacao is more than just a food; it's a lifestyle. Embrace the many ways in which cacao can enrich your life. Incorporate it into your daily routine for its health benefits, use it to enhance your culinary creations, and explore its spiritual and cultural significance. By embracing the cacao lifestyle, you can nourish your body, mind, and spirit and create a life filled with joy, health, and abundance.

The Cacao Manifesto is a call to action for all who believe in the power of cacao to transform our lives and our world. It's a celebration of the rich history, diverse flavors, and incredible potential of this extraordinary bean. So, let's raise a cup of cacao to a chocolate-filled life, one that is delicious, nutritious, sustainable, and joyful.